Table of Contents

Introduction

In the fast-paced world we live in, the quest for holistic health and wellness has never been more prominent. Amidst the myriad of therapeutic practices that have stood the test of time, massage therapy emerges as a beacon of relief, healing, and tranquility. This ancient practice, which spans cultures and millennia, has evolved into a sophisticated tool for enhancing both physical and mental well-being. "The Healing Touch: Unveiling the Benefits of Massage Therapy in Health and Wellness" aims to demystify the art and science of massage therapy, inviting readers into a world where touch holds the power to transform.

The roots of massage therapy stretch deep into history, with its healing touches being one of the earliest forms of medical treatment. From the luxurious spas of ancient Rome to the serene temples of traditional Chinese medicine, massage has been revered as a vital component of health and wellness. Today, it stands at the intersection of traditional wisdom and modern science, offering solutions to the complex health challenges of the contemporary world.

As we peel back the layers of massage therapy, we uncover a multitude of techniques each with its unique benefits. From the gentle strokes of Swedish massage to the targeted pressure of deep tissue work, massage therapy offers a personalized approach to health, ensuring that the needs of the individual are met with precision and care.

The importance of integrating massage into our wellness routines cannot be overstated. In a world where stress is constant and chronic conditions are on the rise, massage therapy offers a refuge—a moment to pause, breathe, and reconnect with our bodies. It invites us to explore the profound impact of touch on our overall well-being, proving that sometimes, the simplest forms of therapy are the most effective.

This book is an invitation to explore the comprehensive benefits of massage therapy. Through its pages, we will journey through the physical, mental, and emotional landscapes of wellness, discovering how massage can play a pivotal role in achieving a balanced, healthy life. Whether you are a seasoned advocate of massage or a curious newcomer, "The Healing Touch" offers insights, evidence, and inspiration to embrace massage therapy as a vital component of your health and wellness strategy. Welcome to the world of massage therapy, where each touch is a step closer to holistic well-being.

Chapter 1

Definition and Types of Massage Therapy:

Massage therapy is an incredible approach to taking care of your body and mind, using the power and simplicity of touch. It goes way beyond just making you feel relaxed and good—it's about therapeutic benefits that target muscle soreness, tension, and even emotional stress.

Imagine your body as this complex network where everything is connected. Sometimes, due to stress, injury, or just everyday activities, this network gets blocked or "knotted up," causing discomfort or pain. Massage therapy comes into play here, acting like a skilled navigator, working through these blockages to restore smooth traffic flow within your body. This isn't just metaphorical; it literally helps improve blood circulation, ensuring oxygen and essential nutrients reach every part of your body more efficiently, aiding in recovery and overall health.

But massage therapy isn't only about the physical perks. It also offers a mental timeout, providing a space where you can disconnect from the outside world and its demands. This mental break can reduce stress levels, improve your mood, and even help with anxiety and depression by promoting a sense of well-being and relaxation.

Therapists use a variety of techniques tailored to what your body needs. Whether it's the gentle strokes of a Swedish massage or the more focused pressure of deep tissue therapy, each method is designed to address specific issues like chronic pain, muscle recovery, or simply stress relief.

Incorporating massage therapy into your wellness routine is like giving your body and mind a comprehensive tune-up. It's a proactive step towards maintaining balance, enhancing physical health, and nurturing mental tranquility. For people dealing with the pressures life throws out, massage therapy can be a valuable tool for managing stress, improving focus, and maintaining physical well-being.

In essence, massage therapy is more than just a luxury or a one-off treat; it's an investment in your holistic health, offering benefits that can support you.

Massage therapy, at its core, is a beautiful and simple way to help your body heal, relax, and feel better using the power of touch. When a massage therapist works on your body, they're not just randomly touching you. They're using specific techniques that have been developed over centuries to target the muscles, tendons, ligaments, skin, and fascia—that's the connective tissue that wraps around everything in your body to keep it all together.

Let's break down how it works:

1. Gentle Stroking (Effleurage): This is like the introduction in a massage. The therapist uses light, smooth strokes with their hands or finger tips over your skin. It's not just for relaxation; it's also to prepare your muscles for deeper work. This technique helps increase blood flow to the area, warming up your muscles and making them more pliable for what's next.

2. Kneading (Petrissage): Imagine someone gently but firmly kneading dough—that's what this feels like on your muscles. The therapist uses their hands to lift, roll, and squeeze your muscles. This goes deeper than effleurage, working out knots and tension in the muscles. It's great for making tight muscles feel looser and more relaxed.

3. Deep Pressure (Deep Tissue): When muscles are really tight or when there's chronic muscle tension, deeper pressure can help. The therapist might use their thumbs, knuckles, or even elbows to apply more force, reaching the deeper layers of muscle and fascia. This technique can really target those stubborn areas of tension, helping to break up knots and restore normal muscle function.

4. Tapping (Tapotement): This technique involves rhythmic tapping or chopping motions on the muscles. It sounds odd, but it's surprisingly relaxing and stimulating at the same time. It can help wake up sleepy muscles, improve circulation, and even help with muscle tone.

5. Friction: Here, the therapist uses pressure along the muscle or across tendons and ligaments to break down adhesions (basically, areas where the tissues are stuck together) and improve mobility. It can be a bit intense, but it's excellent for areas where movement feels restricted because of muscle tightness or scar tissue.

Each of these techniques is applied thoughtfully, taking into account what your body needs. A good massage therapist can feel where there are issues in the muscles or fascia and adjust their technique to help. Whether it's the gentle warmth of effleurage or the focused pressure of deep tissue work, each method has its place in helping your body feel its best.

In massage therapy, the goal is always to support your body's natural ability to heal and maintain itself. By working with the body's tissues in these specific ways, massage can help relieve pain, reduce stress, improve movement, and promote overall well-being. It's a powerful reminder of how something as simple as touch can have such profound effects on our health and happiness.

Massage therapy encompasses a diverse range of techniques, each designed to cater to different health needs and personal preferences. Understanding the main types of massage therapy can help you choose the best approach for your own wellness journey. Here's an overview of some of the most popular forms:

1. **Swedish Massage:** Often considered the most common type of massage, Swedish massage is the foundation for many other types of Western massage. It involves a combination of five basic strokes, all flowing toward the heart, designed to warm up and work the muscle tissues, releasing tension and breaking up muscle "knots." The techniques include effleurage (long, smooth strokes), petrissage (kneading and rolling), tapotement (rhythmic tapping), friction, and vibration or shaking. This type of massage is generally considered ideal for beginners and those looking for a relaxing, therapeutic experience.

2. **Deep Tissue Massage:** As the name suggests, deep tissue massage focuses on the deeper layers of muscle and fascia, the connective tissue surrounding muscles. It uses many of the same movements and techniques as Swedish massage but with more intense pressure to release chronic muscle tension and knots. Deep tissue massage is recommended for individuals who experience consistent pain, are involved in heavy physical activity, or have sustained physical injury.

3. **Sports Massage:** Designed specifically for athletes, sports massage is tailored to the unique needs of sports participants. It focuses on areas of the body that are overused and stressed from repetitive and often

aggressive movements. Sports massage can be used as a means to enhance pre-event preparation and reduce recovery time for maximum performance during an event. It's also used post-event to help heal and rehabilitate injuries.

4. Reflexology: Unlike other types of massage that directly manipulate muscles, reflexology focuses on applying pressure to specific points on the feet, hands, or ears. These points are believed to correspond to different organs and systems in the body. Reflexology is based on the premise that applying pressure to these areas can promote health in the corresponding parts through energetic pathways. It is often sought out for stress relief and for supporting health in related body systems.

Each of these massage therapies offers unique benefits and is suited to particular needs and objectives. Whether you're looking to relax and unwind, alleviate muscle tension, enhance athletic performance, or seek relief from specific health issues, there's a type of massage therapy that can cater to your needs. Understanding these differences is key to choosing the right type of massage for your personal wellness goals, ensuring that you receive the most beneficial and satisfying massage experience.

How Massage Therapy Works: Understanding the Science:

This segment delves into the physiological mechanisms behind massage therapy's effectiveness. It explains how the application of pressure and movement on the body's tissues stimulates blood circulation, facilitates the removal of toxins, reduces muscle tension, and can promote emotional relaxation through the reduction of stress hormones. The explanation extends to how massage activates the body's parasympathetic nervous system, leading to a rest-and-digest response that counteracts the stress-induced fight-or-flight response. This section aims to demystify the science of touch and its profound effects on both the body and mind, reinforcing massage therapy's legitimacy as a therapeutic intervention.

The Role of Massage in the Body's Natural Healing Process:

This part explores how massage therapy complements the body's intrinsic ability to heal itself. It highlights the ways in which massage can accelerate recovery from injuries by enhancing nutrient and oxygen delivery to damaged tissues, facilitating the healing of soft tissue, and reducing inflammation. Additionally, it touches on the psychological benefits of massage, such as the reduction of stress and anxiety, which indirectly contribute to the healing process by improving the overall state of mind and reducing the body's stress responses. This section underscores the holistic impact of massage, showing how it supports both the physical and emotional aspects of healing and wellness.

Chapter 2

Enhancing Circulation and Promoting Tissue Repair:

Massage therapy plays a pivotal role in improving blood circulation throughout the body, which is crucial for promoting healing and overall health. When muscles and tissues are massaged, the physical manipulation has a direct effect on the circulation of blood through the areas being worked on. This enhanced circulation brings a wealth of benefits, crucially including the promotion of healing processes within the body. Here's a deeper look into how massage therapy aids in this vital function:

Enhanced Circulation

During a massage, therapists apply pressure that moves blood through congested or damaged areas, while the release of this pressure causes new blood to flow into tissues. This process helps in removing lactic acid from the muscles and improves the circulation of lymph fluid, which carries metabolic waste away from muscles and internal organs. This results in lower blood pressure levels and an improved overall body function.

Promotion of Healing

With improved circulation, more oxygen and nutrients are delivered to damaged or strained tissues and organs. This influx is crucial for healing, as oxygen is essential for the repair and regeneration of cells. Nutrients, on the other hand, provide the building blocks required for tissue repair. By increasing the flow of these vital components to the areas in need, massage therapy can accelerate the healing process following an injury or relieve conditions caused by poor circulation.

Reducing Swelling and Edema

Massage therapy's ability to enhance blood circulation also helps in reducing swelling and edema (fluid retention) in the body. By encouraging the flow of lymph, which is the body's natural defense system, massage helps in draining excess fluid from the tissues and reducing swelling. This is particularly beneficial after surgery or injury and can also aid individuals suffering from conditions that cause chronic inflammation and edema.

Supporting Cardiovascular Health

Good circulation is foundational to cardiovascular health. By aiding in the efficient flow of blood, massage therapy can help reduce the strain on the heart, potentially lowering blood pressure and improving heart health over time. The relaxation effect of massage also plays a role here, as stress reduction can lead to a decrease in heart rate and blood pressure, further supporting the cardiovascular system.

Facilitating Holistic Healing

Beyond the physical benefits, the improvement in blood circulation also contributes to a holistic sense of well-being. Better circulation means more efficient removal of toxins from the body, improved energy levels, and enhanced mental clarity. The relaxation and stress relief that come from massage therapy further amplify these benefits, creating a positive feedback loop that promotes overall health and wellness.

In conclusion, the role of massage therapy in improving blood circulation is both fundamental and far-reaching. By facilitating the flow of blood, massage therapy not only promotes healing at the site of injury or tension but also supports the body's overall functioning and well-being. This makes massage an invaluable tool in both preventive health care and the recovery process, highlighting the profound impact of this ancient practice on modern-day health.

Improved circulation is crucial for the efficient removal of waste products and detoxification of the body, serving as a cornerstone for maintaining health and preventing disease. When blood circulation is optimized, it not only delivers oxygen and nutrients to cells more effectively but also plays a vital role in the body's natural detoxification process. Here's how this works:

1. Enhanced Blood Flow: The circulatory system is responsible for transporting blood throughout the body. Improved circulation means that blood flows more freely, reaching every part of the body, including the extremities and peripheral areas. This enhanced blood flow carries with it oxygen and vital nutrients that cells need to function and thrive.

2. Removal of Metabolic Wastes: As cells utilize these nutrients, they produce waste products, such as carbon dioxide and urea. Efficient blood circulation ensures that these waste products are promptly carried away from the tissues to the organs responsible for their elimination, such as the kidneys, liver, and lungs. For instance, carbon dioxide is transported to the lungs to be exhaled, while the kidneys filter out urea and other waste products to be expelled in the urine.

3. Lymphatic System Support: The lymphatic system works closely with the circulatory system to remove waste and toxins from the body. Unlike the circulatory system, the lymphatic system does not have a pump like the heart to move lymph fluid throughout the body. Instead, it relies on muscle movement and the pulsing of nearby arteries to propel lymph fluid, which contains waste products and toxins absorbed from the tissues, back into the bloodstream for removal. Improved blood circulation aids in this process by ensuring that the lymphatic system functions more efficiently, thereby enhancing the body's detoxification process.

4. Reducing Edema: Efficient circulation helps prevent the buildup of fluid in the tissues, known as edema, which can result from the accumulation of waste products and toxins. By promoting the removal of these substances, improved circulation helps reduce swelling and supports the overall health of the body's tissues.

5. Stimulating Organ Function: Organs like the liver and kidneys play a crucial role in detoxifying the body. Improved circulation ensures that these organs receive the blood supply they need to perform optimally. For instance, the liver processes toxins and waste products from the blood, transforming them into harmless substances or ensuring they are released from the body. Similarly, the kidneys filter blood to remove waste products and excess fluids. Enhanced circulation supports the efficient functioning of these organs, aiding in the body's natural detoxification processes.

In summary, improved circulation is fundamental to the body's ability to detoxify and eliminate waste. Through the enhanced delivery of oxygen and nutrients and the efficient removal of metabolic waste products, a well-functioning circulatory system supports the health and proper functioning of every cell, tissue, and organ in the body, contributing to overall well-being and the prevention of disease.

Pain Relief: Managing Chronic Pain and Acute Injuries

Massage therapy has emerged as a formidable ally in the management of both chronic pain and acute injuries, offering a non-invasive, holistic approach to pain relief. Unlike pharmacological treatments, which often come with side effects and the potential for dependency, massage therapy provides a safe, natural alternative for alleviating pain, highlighting its importance in both preventive care and rehabilitation.

Understanding Pain and the Body's Response

At its core, pain is a complex and subjective experience, influenced by a myriad of physical, emotional, and psychological factors. Chronic pain, defined as pain persisting for more than three months, can stem from ongoing health conditions, such as arthritis or fibromyalgia, or as a result of unresolved injuries. Acute pain, on the other hand, is a sudden, sharp sensation signaling tissue damage or injury. Massage therapy addresses both types by engaging the body's natural healing mechanisms, promoting a sense of wellness and relief.

The Mechanisms Behind Massage Therapy's Effectiveness

Massage therapy reduces pain through several physiological processes. By manipulating soft tissues, massage encourages blood flow to the affected areas, delivering oxygen and essential nutrients that facilitate the healing of tissues. This improved circulation helps flush out toxins and metabolic waste from muscle fibers, reducing inflammation and the accompanying pain.

Furthermore, massage therapy works on a neurological level. It interrupts pain signaling pathways to the brain, a process known as the "gate control theory" of pain. By stimulating nerves that do not transmit pain signals, massage can effectively "close the gate" on pain messages, offering immediate relief. Additionally, massage therapy increases the production of endorphins, the body's natural painkillers, and serotonin, a neurotransmitter associated with feelings of well-being and decreased pain perception.

Addressing Specific Conditions

For individuals suffering from chronic conditions like arthritis, massage therapy can be particularly beneficial. By enhancing joint flexibility and reducing stiffness, it can lead to significant reductions in pain and discomfort, improving quality of life. Similarly, for those recovering from acute injuries, such as sports-related strains or sprains, massage can speed up the recovery process by reducing swelling and preventing the formation of excessive scar tissue, which can lead to long-term mobility issues.

Massage therapy also proves effective in managing pain from tension-related conditions, such as headaches and migraines. By targeting the muscles of the neck, shoulders, and head, it can alleviate the tension that often triggers these painful episodes.

Customizing the Approach

One of the key strengths of massage therapy in pain management lies in its adaptability. Therapists can tailor their techniques to the specific needs and conditions of each individual, choosing from a variety of modalities such as Swedish massage for general relaxation and pain relief, deep tissue massage for chronic muscle tension, or trigger point therapy for localized pain relief.

Empowering Patients

Beyond its direct effects on pain, massage therapy empowers individuals to play an active role in their healing process. It provides a therapeutic pause from the stresses of daily life, encouraging a deeper connection with one's body. This mindfulness aspect can enhance the perception of pain relief and promote a more profound sense of well-being.

In conclusion, massage therapy stands as a pivotal component of integrative health care for pain management. Its ability to address pain from multiple angles—not just the physical symptoms but also the emotional and psychological aspects—makes it an invaluable tool in the pursuit of health and wellness. By incorporating massage therapy into their care regimen, individuals can discover a path to not only managing pain but also enhancing their overall quality of life, proving that sometimes, the most ancient practices hold the keys to modern health challenges.

Improving Flexibility and Range of Motion

Alright, let's get this straight—when we talk about improving flexibility and range of motion, we're essentially trying to ensure you don't sound like a creaky door every time you bend down. Yes, I'm looking at you, the one who groans louder than an old floorboard when picking up something off the ground. Massage therapy is here to turn you from a stiff board into a bendy straw, and trust me, it's less about turning into a pretzel and more about ensuring you can tie your shoelaces without issuing a public service announcement.

Why Flexibility Is No Joke

Flexibility might seem like something reserved for circus performers or those freaky folks who enjoy twisting themselves into human knots for fun. But here's the kicker: being flexible is actually about making everyday life less of a hassle. Imagine reaching for that top shelf without feeling like you're auditioning for a role in "The Hunchback of Notre Dame." That's the dream, folks. And massage therapy? It's your secret weapon.

The Science of Stretching

Now, onto the science bit—bear with me, it's not as dry as it sounds. When a massage therapist gets their hands on you, they're doing more than just making you feel like you're being kneaded like pizza dough. They're working out those knots and tension spots that make your muscles as pliable as a two-by-four. The process increases blood flow, which is like sending a VIP invite to oxygen and nutrients to come party in your muscles, making them more elastic and less like they're made of concrete.

Bend It Like... You?

Here's the deal: improving your flexibility and range of motion isn't just about bragging rights at yoga class or impressing someone with your sudden ability to kick higher than your head (although, admittedly, that's pretty cool). It's about reducing the risk of injuries, because let's face it, pulling a muscle while reaching for the remote is both embarrassing and entirely preventable. Massage therapy helps you achieve that "bend, don't break" philosophy in a literal sense.

The Chronicles of Stiff-as-a-Board to Limber Larry

So, you start your journey resembling something akin to a medieval knight in full armor—rigid, noble, and not particularly bendy. Enter massage therapy: the heroic squire ready to loosen up those joints and muscles with the magic of touch (and a bit of elbow grease). Before you know it, you're moving with the grace of a slightly awkward swan, but hey, progress is progress!

Flexibility: The Gift That Keeps on Giving

As your flexibility improves, so does your life. You'll find joy in simple things, like sneezing without fearing a muscle spasm, or actually enjoying activities that used to seem like torture. Suddenly, putting on socks becomes a moment of triumph rather than a battle of wills. Plus, your newfound range of motion means you can wave goodbye to people with such flair that you might just start doing it for fun.

In conclusion, while we've had our laughs, let's not forget that improving flexibility and range of motion is genuinely beneficial, and massage therapy is your not-so-secret weapon in achieving that. So, get ready to bend the rules (and yourself) in ways you never thought possible, and remember: life's too short to be stiff.

Enhancing Flexibility and Range of Motion: A Gentle Journey to Movement and Grace

In the tapestry of wellness, the threads of flexibility and range of motion are woven with the utmost care and affection. Imagine a world where each movement is fluid, each stretch a whisper of freedom. This isn't just the domain of dancers or athletes; it's a reachable reality for each of us, thanks to the nurturing touch of massage therapy. As we embark on this gentle journey, let's explore how massage can be a tender companion in enhancing our body's grace and vitality.

A Tender Touch for Taut Muscles

Our bodies, these incredible vessels of life and experience, sometimes hold onto tension like cherished keepsakes. Over time, this tension can limit our movement, making us feel like we're wearing a suit of armor we never asked for. Massage therapy, with its caring touch, works to unlock this armor. Through skilled hands, a massage therapist can coax muscles into releasing their grip, inviting flexibility and range of motion to return like birds to springtime trees.

The Art of Listening to Our Bodies

In our bustling lives, it's easy to forget the art of stillness, of truly listening to the whispers of our bodies. Massage therapy offers a pause, a quiet moment to connect with ourselves. It reminds us that caring for our bodies is not just about doing but also about being. As we lie on the massage table, we're not just being treated; we're being taught — taught to honor our limitations, to gently push against them, and to celebrate the smallest expansions of movement.

A Journey Together

Enhancing flexibility isn't a solitary endeavor but a shared journey with your massage therapist. They become your guide, understanding your body's unique story, its silent aches, and its aspirations for freedom. Together, you navigate the path toward greater movement, each session a step further along the road of well-being. This partnership, built on trust and understanding, becomes a powerful force for healing and growth.

The Ripple Effects of a Flexible Body

As flexibility and range of motion begin to blossom, so too does the rest of our lives. Activities that once seemed daunting become sources of joy. A morning stretch transforms into a moment of gratitude. We find beauty in the ability to reach further, not just physically, but in all aspects of our lives. This newfound grace is not confined to the yoga mat or the dance floor; it permeates every step, every gesture, imbuing our daily routines with a sense of ease and joy.

Caring Beyond the Massage Table

The journey to enhanced flexibility doesn't end at the massage therapist's door. They equip us with the knowledge and techniques to continue caring for our bodies at home. Simple stretches, mindful movements, and the practice of listening to our bodies become part of our daily ritual. This self-care is a testament to the respect and love we owe ourselves, ensuring that the benefits of massage extend far beyond the session.

In closing, enhancing flexibility and range of motion through massage therapy is much more than a physical transformation. It's a journey of reconnection with our bodies, led by the caring hands of a therapist who reminds us of the beauty in movement. As we embrace this gentle path, let us carry with us the knowledge that to care for our bodies is to honor the very essence of life itself.

Stress Reduction and Management: A Compassionate Guide to Inner Peace

In the tapestry of life, stress often weaves its intricate patterns, sometimes overshadowing the vibrant hues of joy and tranquility. Yet, amidst this complex interplay, massage therapy emerges as a gentle, nurturing force, capable of softening the harsh lines of stress and guiding us toward a state of inner peace. This chapter is a tender exploration of how the caring touch of massage can be a sanctuary for the weary soul, offering a respite from the storms of life and nurturing the seeds of calm within.

A Sanctuary of Calm

Imagine, if you will, a place where the relentless pace of life slows, where the burdens of the mind gently lift, leaving a space for tranquility to bloom. This is the essence of stress reduction through massage therapy. It is not merely a physical relief but a journey to a mental and emotional oasis. The power of touch, so fundamental yet profound, speaks a language of compassion and understanding, telling our bodies and minds that it is safe to release the grip of stress.

The Art of Mindful Presence

In the realm of massage therapy, each stroke and knead is an invitation to mindfulness, a gentle call to anchor ourselves in the present moment. This practice of being fully engaged in the now, with each breath and touch, is a powerful antidote to stress. It encourages a dialogue between body and mind, one that fosters a deep sense of calm and awareness. This mindfulness, nurtured on the massage table, can ripple out into everyday life, offering tools to manage stress with grace and poise.

The Healing Power of Connection

At its heart, the reduction of stress through massage is about connection—connection to oneself, to the therapist, and to the universal need for care and understanding. This connection reaffirms our shared humanity, reminding us that we are not alone in our struggles. The therapist's touch becomes a bridge, crossing the distances we sometimes feel within ourselves, reconnecting us to our essence and to the comforting truth that peace is within reach.

A Compassionate Journey

As we embark on this journey of stress reduction, let us do so with kindness towards ourselves. Let the massage table be a place of release and discovery, where the layers of tension melt away to reveal the calm, resilient self that resides within. Through the compassionate art of massage therapy, we learn not just to manage stress, but to embrace the possibility of a life lived with serenity and grace.

In embracing this path, we find that the greatest strength lies in gentleness, and the truest form of peace begins with a compassionate touch.

Chapter 3

The Magic Touch: How Massage Magically Melts Away Your Stress

Alright, folks, let's dive into the wonderfully squishy world of massage therapy, where the only homework is to relax, and the only test is whether you can stay awake long enough to enjoy it. It's a tough job, but hey, someone's gotta do it!

The Stress Monster and Its Favorite Snack: You

Let's face it, life can sometimes feel like you're the main character in a video game set to "impossible" difficulty. Homework, exams, social drama—it's like stress has a personal vendetta against you. But fear not, dear reader, for there is a hero in this tale, and it's not a knight in shining armor but a knight with magic hands: the massage therapist.

Why Massage, You Ask?

Imagine your body is a city, Stressville, where traffic jams are made of tight muscles and the citizens are as tense as a finals week. Now, imagine a superhero sweeping in, not with a cape, but with a bottle of massage oil and hands that could make even the grumpiest muscles purr like a kitten. That's massage therapy for you.

The Science of Chill

So, how does this magical transformation happen? When a massage therapist goes to work, they're not just making you feel like you're floating on a cloud of bliss for the fun of it (though that is a pretty great side effect). They're kicking your body's relaxation response into high gear, telling your brain to chill out and your muscles to take a much-needed vacation.

Massage boosts your body's production of the feel-good squad: endorphins, serotonin, and dopamine, while giving the stress hormone cortisol a time-out. It's like your body's version of switching from a horror movie to a comedy.

The Ripple Effect of Relaxation

But wait, there's more! Not only does massage make your muscles feel like they've just come back from a spa vacation, but it also helps you sleep better, focus more, and might even make that history test seem less like a battle and more like a mildly amusing quiz show.

A Touch of Humor

Remember, while massage can work wonders, it's also okay to laugh if you find yourself snoring on the table or drooling on the pillow. It's all part of the stress-relief process. And let's be honest, is there anything more relaxing than a good laugh?

So, next time you're feeling like you're about to be crowned the monarch of Stressville, consider booking a trip to your local massage therapist. It's one vacation where you don't have to pack a thing, and the souvenirs—peace of mind and a rejuvenated body—are priceless.

In conclusion, if life's got you in knots, a massage is the perfect way to tie up those loose ends. So, take a deep breath, book that appointment, and prepare to laugh in the face of stress. After all, in the battle of You vs. Stress, you've got the ultimate secret weapon: the magic touch of massage.

Massage Help for Anxiety and Depression

In the grand adventure of life, where anxiety and depression can sometimes feel like uninvited guests crashing your soul's party, there's a gentle warrior ready to help you show these party poopers the door: massage therapy. Yes, that's right, the ancient art of pressing, kneading, and gliding over sore muscles can actually be a beacon of light in the fog of mental health struggles. So, grab a cup of tea, snuggle into your coziest blanket, and let's explore how this touchy-feely ally fights off the blues and the mean reds with compassion, humor, and some pretty impressive science.

The Power of Touch

Imagine your nervous system as a highly strung musical instrument, always on the verge of playing a sour note at the slightest provocation. Now, enter massage therapy: the skilled maestro ready to tune that instrument to the harmonious sound of relaxation. This isn't just about making your muscles feel like well-kneaded dough; it's about communicating safety, care, and support through the universal language of touch. It's a kind reminder that you're not alone, turning touch into a powerful message of healing.

The Chemical Cocktail Party

Your body, bless its heart, is like a walking, talking chemistry lab, constantly mixing up concoctions that affect how you feel. When anxiety and depression are the unwanted guests at the party, massage therapy steps in like a master mixologist, changing the vibe by adjusting the chemical playlist. It reduces cortisol, the stress DJ that never knows when to quit, and boosts serotonin and dopamine, the life of the party, ensuring your body's chemical cocktail promotes feelings of well-being, happiness, and relaxation.

The Art of Breathing Easy

Ever noticed how, when you're anxious or down, your breaths become short and choppy, as if you're preparing to blow out a thousand birthday candles with one breath? Massage therapy introduces a change in tempo, inviting deep, slow breaths that tell your body, "Hey, it's okay. You've got this." This not only oxygenates your brain and muscles but also conducts the orchestra of your inner systems to play a soothing symphony of calm.

Laughter: The Best Medicine (After Massage)

Let's not forget the power of laughter. While massage gets to work on your muscles, let's tickle your funny bone with the idea that you're essentially paying someone to give you a glorified hug and make you feel wonderful. It's like ordering a side of happiness with your main course of relaxation. And if the thought of accidentally drooling or snoring mid-massage makes you blush, remember that in the realm of massage therapy, these are just the body's own quirky ways of saying, "Thank you, I needed that."

A Compassionate Ally in Your Corner

In the end, massage therapy is more than just a temporary escape from the weight of the world. It's a compassionate ally, whispering to every cell of your being that it's okay to take a moment for yourself, to heal, and to find peace amidst the chaos. It's a reminder that, just like in the movies, good things come to those who reach out for help, even if that help comes in the form of a massage table and some soothing oils.

So, if anxiety and depression are gatecrashing your mental peace, consider massage therapy as your kindly bouncer, ready to show them out and invite relaxation, laughter, and a renewed sense of well-being. Remember, in the dance of life, you deserve to lead with joy.

I just want to sleep. . .

In the gentle journey towards a night of peaceful slumber, massage therapy emerges as a kind and caring guide, leading you through the twists and turns of restlessness to the serene destination of deep, restorative sleep. It's like having a friend who whispers, "Relax, I've got you," as they guide you through a darkened path, ensuring each step is taken with care and comfort.

The Warm Embrace of Relaxation

Think of your body as a sanctuary that, after a long day, deserves to unwind and be free of the day's burdens. Massage acts like a gentle custodian of this sanctuary, easing the tension and stress that cling to your muscles like unwelcome shadows, casting them away with every stroke and knead. This physical release is the body's way of letting go, signaling that it's time to move from the hustle and bustle of the day into the soft, soothing embrace of the night.

A Lullaby for Your Nervous System

Your nervous system, that intricate network of signals and responses, can sometimes get stuck in 'alert' mode, making it hard to settle down. Massage whispers a calming lullaby to this vigilant guardian, soothing it into a state of restful alertness. This lullaby lowers the heart rate, relaxes the breath, and prepares the body for sleep, much like a parent soothing a child to sleep with gentle back rubs and quiet reassurances.

The Dream Weavers Toolkit

As the massage eases your body into relaxation, it also encourages the release of serotonin, a key player in the production of melatonin, the body's own sleep hormone. Think of serotonin as the dream weaver's thread, delicately stitching together the fabric of your sleep. With each massage, you're adding more thread, weaving a tapestry of dreams that cradle you through the night.

The Nightly Ritual of Self-Care

Incorporating massage into your routine becomes a ritual of self-care, a reminder that you are worthy of kindness and nurturing. This ritual helps set the stage for sleep, creating a sanctuary not just in your physical space but within yourself. It's a practice that says, "This time is for me," allowing you to honor the natural rhythms of your body and mind, and to embrace the night with a sense of peace and readiness for sleep.

A Journey of Gentle Discovery

For those who find the night elusive, massage offers a path of gentle discovery, exploring what it means to truly relax and let go. It's an invitation to deepen your relationship with your body, to listen to its needs, and to respond with kindness and care. As you journey towards better sleep, you learn to carry this kindness with you, letting it infuse your nights with tranquility and your days with calm.

In the embrace of massage therapy, sleep becomes more than just a necessity; it becomes a cherished friend, eagerly awaited and warmly welcomed. So, as you lay down tonight, remember the gentle power of massage to guide you to the land of dreams, where rest and rejuvenation await with open arms.

How massage helps mood and clarity

Embarking on a journey to understand how massage boosts mood and mental clarity is like delving into a beautiful, intricate dance between the body and mind. This dance, grounded in both the art of touch and the science of healing, reveals the profound impact of massage on our emotional and cognitive well-being. With kindness at its core, let's explore the science behind this nurturing touch and its capacity to clear the mind and elevate the spirit.

The Biochemical Ballet

At the heart of massage therapy's ability to enhance mood lies a delicate biochemical ballet. As hands glide over the body, they do more than simply relax tense muscles; they activate a complex physiological response that orchestrates a shift in the body's chemistry. This response includes the reduction of cortisol, the body's primary stress hormone. High levels of cortisol are associated with stress, anxiety, and depression, so its reduction through massage can lead to an immediate feeling of relief and calm.

Simultaneously, massage encourages the release of endorphins, serotonin, and dopamine—neurotransmitters that play starring roles in our feelings of happiness and well-being. Endorphins, often referred to as the body's natural painkillers, not only alleviate pain but also induce feelings of pleasure and euphoria. Serotonin regulates mood, combating feelings of depression, while dopamine enhances focus and motivation, contributing to a sense of clarity and purpose. Together, these chemical messengers perform a harmonious symphony that lifts the mood and sharpens the mind.

The Physical Connection to Emotional Well-being

The physical benefits of massage—such as reduced muscle tension and improved blood circulation—also contribute to its mood-enhancing effects. By relieving physical discomfort, massage can help remove physical barriers to mental clarity. Improved circulation ensures that more oxygen and nutrients are delivered to the brain, which can lead to better cognitive function and a clearer mind. Furthermore, the act of touch itself can be incredibly powerful. Human touch is a fundamental need, promoting feelings of safety, trust, and connection. When we receive a massage, we experience a nurturing form of touch that can be deeply comforting and reassuring, reinforcing a sense of well-being and emotional balance.

Creating a Space for Healing and Reflection

Massage provides a unique opportunity for quiet reflection and mindfulness. In the tranquil space created by the therapist's touch, the mind is encouraged to pause and disengage from the constant chatter and distractions of daily life. This mental break can foster an environment where clarity and creativity flourish, and where emotional burdens can be viewed from a new perspective, facilitating healing and emotional resilience.

A Cycle of Renewal

The benefits of massage extend beyond the immediate post-massage glow. Regular massage therapy can help establish a more sustained cycle of mood enhancement and mental clarity. Over time, this can lead to improved stress management, better sleep patterns, and a more positive outlook on life. By integrating massage into our self-care routine, we are investing in our long-term emotional and cognitive health, reinforcing a cycle of renewal and well-being.

In the gentle, caring hands of massage therapy, we find a powerful ally in our quest for emotional balance and mental clarity. Through the science of its healing touch, massage offers a pathway to a brighter mood and a clearer mind, wrapped in the kindness and compassion that we all deserve.

Chapter 4

When we think of fortifying our immune system, we often turn to the familiar allies of nutrition, exercise, and sufficient sleep. Yet, there's another, perhaps more gentle and compassionate ally in this quest for well-being: massage therapy. Through the power of touch, massage not only offers a soothing embrace to the body and soul but also actively engages and strengthens our body's natural defenses. Let's explore this nurturing path to enhanced immunity with both the heart and the science in mind.

A Tender Touch Against Stress

At its core, massage therapy acts as a powerful countermeasure to stress, a known adversary of the immune system. Chronic stress puts the body in a constant state of "fight or flight," which can lead to inflammation and weaken the immune response. Massage, with its inherent ability to reduce stress and promote relaxation, helps to calm this response. By lowering levels of cortisol and increasing the production of serotonin, massage not only soothes the stressed spirit but also supports the body's ability to fend off pathogens. Imagine each stroke of the massage as a gentle reminder to your body that it's time to shift from a state of alertness to one of rest and repair, allowing your immune cells to perform at their best.

The Lymphatic System's Gentle Encouragement

The lymphatic system, a crucial component of our immune system, relies on movement and muscle action to transport lymph—a fluid containing white blood cells and waste products—throughout the body. Massage assists this process by encouraging the flow of lymph, effectively supporting the body's natural detoxification process and enhancing the function of the immune system. This is akin to gently clearing the paths in a garden, allowing nourishment to reach the plants more effectively and waste to be removed efficiently, thus ensuring the garden's health and vitality.

Enhanced Circulation, Enhanced Vigilance

Improved blood circulation is another gift of massage to the body, with a direct impact on immune health. Enhanced circulation means that oxygen and nutrients are more efficiently delivered to tissues and organs, including those involved in the immune response. This not only aids in the repair and renewal of the body but also ensures that immune cells are distributed more effectively throughout the body. It's as if massage ensures that the sentinels of our immune system can patrol more widely and diligently, keeping watch over our health with greater vigilance.

A Sanctuary for Healing

Beyond the physical benefits, the act of receiving a massage creates a sanctuary where emotional and physical healing can coexist. This sanctuary is a place of comfort and rest, where the psychological burden of illness or stress can be momentarily lifted, allowing the immune system to function without additional psychological stressors. In this space, the body finds a haven of peace, reminding us of the interconnectedness of our emotional well-being and physical health.

A Compassionate Partnership

Viewing massage as a partner in our journey towards health offers a compassionate perspective on self-care. It's a practice that acknowledges the body's innate wisdom and its ability to heal when given support and care. Regular massage therapy can be a testament to the commitment to nurture oneself, reinforcing the body's resilience and our dedication to maintaining our health.

In embracing massage therapy, we welcome a compassionate ally in our pursuit of a strong immune system. It's a path that honors the body's complexities and its capacity for renewal, inviting us to experience the profound benefits of nurturing touch in our quest for health and well-being.

The lymphatic system and massage

Imagine your body as a bustling city, with streets and pathways for transportation. The lymphatic system is like a special network of waterways that helps to keep the city clean by removing waste and toxins. This system doesn't have a pump, like the heart in your circulatory system, so sometimes it needs a little help to move things along.

Massage steps in as a helpful friend, gently encouraging the movement of lymph fluid through these waterways. By applying smooth, light strokes in the direction that the lymph flows (towards the heart), massage helps to push the lymph fluid forward. Think of it as gently guiding a boat down the river, helping it to navigate and reach its destination more efficiently.

This gentle guidance helps to speed up the removal of waste products and toxins from your body's tissues. It's like clearing traffic jams and blockages in the city's waterways, allowing for a smoother and cleaner environment. As a result, the body can detoxify more effectively, leading to a feeling of refreshment and well-being, much like how a clean and well-maintained city feels more vibrant and healthy.

So, in simple terms, massage helps your lymphatic system work better, aiding in detoxification and keeping your body feeling clean and rejuvenated. It's a natural and soothing way to support your body's own cleansing processes.
Massage might just be your body's very own superhero in disguise, cape and all, when it comes to fending off those pesky villains—illnesses and infections!

First off, let's set the stage with a bit of science, shall we? Imagine your immune system as the city's defense force against the never-ending parade of germs and viruses looking to crash your body's party. Now, massage, in this delightful tale, plays the role of the wise old sage, quietly boosting the ranks of your immune system's soldiers, making them more effective in their battle against the dark forces of sickness.

Massage has been shown to reduce levels of cortisol, the notorious stress hormone that often plays the role of the double agent, weakening the immune system's defenses from the inside. By lowering cortisol levels, massage helps ensure that your immune system is not sabotaging its own efforts, keeping it ready and alert for any invasions.

So, in a world where stress and anxiety lurk around every corner, armed with their trusty sidekicks, colds and flu, massage steps in like a superhero, albeit a very gentle and non-threatening one, perhaps more akin to a superhero whose power is giving really reassuring hugs. It boosts your body's internal defense team, making you less likely to fall victim to the sinister plots of germs and viruses.

In conclusion, while we can't say massage will make you invincible (sadly, you won't be able to leap tall buildings in a single bound), it can be an ally in your quest for health, reducing your susceptibility to illness by keeping your immune system fit and vigilant—like a well-oiled machine, or better yet, a well-massaged superhero ready for action!

Chapter 5

Swedish massage, one of the most popular and widely practiced forms of massage therapy, is renowned for its effectiveness in promoting relaxation and alleviating pain. This method employs a variety of techniques designed to relax muscles by applying pressure against deeper muscles and bones and rubbing in the same direction as the flow of blood returning to the heart. The benefits of Swedish massage extend beyond simple relaxation, encompassing a range of health advantages that contribute to a holistic sense of well-being.

The foundational techniques of Swedish massage include effleurage (long, smooth strokes), petrissage (kneading, rolling, and squeezing), tapotement (rhythmic tapping), friction (firm, circular rubbing motions), and vibration or shaking. Each technique serves a specific purpose in the massage process:

Effleurage: This technique is often used to begin the session, warming up the muscles and encouraging the flow of blood and lymphatic fluids. It sets the stage for deeper work while promoting a state of mental calm.

Petrissage: By lifting and rolling the muscles, petrissage aids in the breakdown of knots and tension in the muscle fibers. This technique enhances muscle flexibility and can significantly reduce pain in areas with accumulated stress.

Tapotement: The rhythmic tapping not only invigorates the body but also stimulates nerve endings, which can boost muscle relaxation and pain relief. It's particularly beneficial for awakening dormant muscles.

Friction: Applied with deep pressure to areas with adhesions or chronic muscle tension, friction generates heat that increases blood circulation, promoting healing and reducing pain.

Vibration/Shaking: These movements help to loosen the muscles and stimulate blood flow, further enhancing relaxation and pain alleviation.

Relaxation and Stress Reduction

Swedish massage directly impacts the nervous system through touch. The gentle, rhythmic strokes activate parasympathetic nervous responses, reducing cortisol levels (stress hormones) and increasing levels of serotonin and dopamine (neurotransmitters associated with happiness and well-being). This biochemical change fosters deep relaxation, reduces stress, and enhances mood, creating a profound sense of overall well-being.

Pain Relief

The increased circulation promoted by Swedish massage techniques delivers oxygen-rich blood to muscle tissues, helping to flush out toxins, reduce swelling, and improve flexibility. This not only accelerates the healing process of injured or overused muscles but also provides relief from chronic pain conditions such as fibromyalgia and arthritis. By addressing the source of the pain, Swedish massage can reduce reliance on medication, offering a natural pain management solution.

Swedish massage offers a therapeutic avenue for relaxation and pain relief, engaging both the body and mind in a healing process. Its gentle yet effective techniques can significantly improve an individual's quality of life, making it a valuable tool for anyone seeking to enhance their well-being through natural, non-invasive means. Whether you're coping with stress, suffering from chronic pain, or simply in need of a moment of tranquility, Swedish massage provides a comprehensive solution that nurtures both physical and emotional health.

Deep tissue massage, a technique that focuses on the deeper layers of muscle and connective tissue, is a therapeutic intervention designed to alleviate muscle tension and address the symptoms associated with chronic illnesses. This form of massage therapy employs sustained pressure using slow, deep strokes to target the inner layers of your muscles and connective tissues. By doing so, it helps to break up scar tissue that forms following an injury and reduce tension in muscle and tissue. It also promotes faster healing by increasing blood flow and reducing inflammation.

Mechanism of Action

The primary mechanism through which deep tissue massage exerts its effects is by the manipulation of soft tissues, which includes muscles, connective tissue, tendons, ligaments, and fascia. The applied pressure helps to physically break down adhesions or bands of painful, rigid tissue in muscles, tendons, and ligaments. Adhesions can block circulation, cause pain, limit movement, and lead to inflammation. By realigning deeper layers of muscles and connective tissue, deep tissue massage is effective in restoring normal movement and reducing pain.

Impact on Muscle Tension

Muscle tension often results from chronic stress and repetitive use injuries, leading to the formation of knots (trigger points) that are painful to the touch. Deep tissue massage works by applying intense pressure to these knots, thereby facilitating muscle relaxation. This technique is particularly beneficial for individuals with chronic muscle tension in areas such as the neck, lower back, and shoulders. Through the specific targeting of affected areas, deep tissue massage can significantly reduce the tightness and discomfort associated with muscle tension, thereby enhancing flexibility and overall physical function.

Role in Managing Chronic Illness

Chronic illnesses, especially those characterized by pain and inflammation, such as fibromyalgia, chronic fatigue syndrome, and arthritis, can benefit from deep tissue massage. By improving circulation, this form of massage therapy aids in the reduction of inflammation and the enhancement of oxygen and nutrient delivery to affected areas. This not only alleviates pain but also supports the body's natural healing processes. Furthermore, the stress relief associated with massage therapy can have a positive impact on individuals with chronic illnesses, contributing to a reduction in the overall burden of disease. The psychological benefits, including reduced symptoms of anxiety and depression, further underscore the holistic impact of deep tissue massage on chronic illness management.

Deep tissue massage represents a valuable therapeutic tool in the management of muscle tension and chronic illness. Through its targeted approach to addressing the deeper layers of muscle and connective tissue, it offers a non-invasive means of pain relief, improved mobility, and enhanced quality of life for individuals suffering from a range of chronic conditions. The physiological and psychological benefits of deep tissue massage underscore its potential as a complementary therapy in the comprehensive management of chronic illnesses, warranting further exploration and integration into holistic health care practices.

Sports massage, a specialized form of massage therapy, is designed with the athlete in mind, from the weekend jogger to the professional competitor. It is a compassionate approach to ensuring that individuals who love to stay active can do so with less pain, more enjoyment, and a lower risk of injury. This therapeutic intervention serves a dual purpose: preparing the body for physical activity and aiding in the recovery process afterward. Let's explore how sports massage benefits those dedicated to their active lifestyles.

Preparing for Activity

Before you embark on any physical endeavor, be it a marathon, a soccer game, or a challenging hike, sports massage can serve as a nurturing preparation for your body. By focusing on the muscles that will be most engaged, sports massage helps to warm and stretch muscle tissue, increasing flexibility and range of motion. This preparation is not just physical; it also mentally prepares you for the upcoming activity. It's a moment of quietude and focus, where you can center yourself, aligning body and mind for the challenges ahead. Think of it as a loving reminder that taking care of your body before pushing its limits is not just prudent; it's an act of self-respect.

Enhancing Performance

During the activity, the benefits of your pre-event sports massage continue to manifest. The increased flexibility and circulation can lead to improved performance, as your body is in a better state to handle the demands placed upon it. This isn't about pushing harder but moving more efficiently, with grace and power, thanks to a body that's been attentively prepared.

Recovery After Activities

After the exertion, sports massage plays a crucial role in the recovery process. It's a compassionate response to the stress and strain your body has endured. By focusing on muscles that have been heavily used, sports massage helps to alleviate the buildup of lactic acid, which can lead to stiffness and soreness. It encourages the flow of fresh blood to these areas, bringing with it oxygen and nutrients that aid in the healing process. This not only accelerates recovery time but also deeply respects the hard work your body has done, acknowledging it with care and attention.

Reducing the Risk of Injury

Regular sports massage can significantly reduce the risk of injury by maintaining the health and elasticity of the muscle tissue. It's a proactive approach, identifying and addressing potential issues before they develop into injuries. This aspect of sports massage is a testament to its role not just in physical maintenance but in injury prevention, underscoring the philosophy that taking care of oneself is the foundation of continued activity and enjoyment of life's physical challenges.

Emotional and Psychological Benefits

Beyond the physical benefits, sports massage offers emotional and psychological relief, reducing stress and anxiety associated with competitions and performance. It's a moment to breathe, to be present, and to feel genuinely cared for. This mental and emotional support is integral to overall wellness and can enhance the joy and satisfaction derived from physical activity.

Sports massage is a deeply compassionate practice, supporting individuals in their pursuit of activity and excellence. It acknowledges the dedication required to stay active and responds with a nurturing touch that prepares, heals, and respects the athlete in everyone. Whether you're gearing up for a big event or winding down from one, sports massage is a valuable ally in your journey toward health, well-being, and the joy of movement.

Reflexology is a holistic healing technique that involves applying pressure to specific points on the feet, hands, and ears, which are believed to correspond to different parts of the body. The theory behind reflexology rests on the concept of zones and reflex areas that map to various organs, glands, and systems of the body. By stimulating these points, reflexologists aim to promote health and well-being throughout the entire body, encouraging balance and natural healing processes.

Theory Behind Reflexology

The foundational theory of reflexology is rooted in the belief that the body is divided into ten vertical zones, running from the top of the head to the tips of the toes and the hands. Each zone corresponds to fingers, toes, and thus to specific body organs and systems within these zones. Reflexologists use this zone theory to target areas of the body that are out of balance or in need of healing, by applying pressure to the related reflex area on the foot, hand, or ear.

How Reflexology Affects the Whole Body

1. Stress Reduction and Relaxation: One of the most immediate effects of reflexology is a deep sense of relaxation. By reducing stress and tension, reflexology encourages the body to shift from a state of fight-or-flight to a state of rest and repair, known as the parasympathetic response. This shift promotes overall healing and is foundational to maintaining balance in the body.

2. Improved Circulation: Reflexology can help improve blood circulation throughout the body, ensuring that oxygen and nutrients are efficiently delivered to all cells. Better circulation aids in the removal of toxins and increases the efficiency of organ function, which in turn can improve health and vitality.

3. Pain Reduction: Through the application of pressure on specific reflex points, reflexology is thought to reduce pain by stimulating the nervous system to release endorphins, the body's natural painkillers. It's particularly noted for its effectiveness in managing headaches, menstrual cramps, and chronic pain conditions.

4. Enhanced Detoxification: Reflexology supports the body's detoxification processes by improving lymphatic flow and

circulation. This can help in flushing out toxins and waste products, potentially reducing inflammation and stimulating the immune system.

5. Balancing the Body's Systems: Reflexology is based on the principle of homeostasis, or balance, within the body. By stimulating points associated with various organs and systems, reflexologists aim to correct imbalances and encourage the body's natural healing capabilities. This can help in addressing specific health issues such as digestive problems, hormonal imbalances, or respiratory conditions.

The theory behind reflexology posits that the body is interconnected, with reflex points on the feet, hands, and ears serving as gateways to promote health and balance throughout the entire organism. By engaging these points, reflexology seeks not only to alleviate symptoms but to address the root causes of imbalance, supporting the body's innate healing processes. While reflexology should not be used as a substitute for medical treatment, it can be a valuable complementary therapy, offering a non-invasive, holistic approach to health and wellness.

Shiatsu and Thai massage are two distinct forms of bodywork that originate from different parts of Asia, each with its unique theory and practice. While they share the common goal of promoting health and well-being by balancing the body's energy, their techniques, and underlying philosophies differ significantly.

Shiatsu

Description: Shiatsu, which literally translates to "finger pressure" in Japanese, is a form of massage that involves applying pressure to specific points on the body. Practitioners use their thumbs, fingers, and palms to apply pressure to areas of the body that are believed to be important for the flow of Qi (vital energy). Shiatsu is performed with the recipient fully clothed, typically on a mat on the floor.

Theory: The theory behind Shiatsu is rooted in traditional Chinese medicine and the concept of Qi. According to this theory, health is a state of balance in which Qi flows freely throughout the body. Illness or discomfort is believed to result from blockages or imbalances in this flow. Shiatsu aims to remove these blockages and restore balance to the body's energy pathways, known as meridians. By stimulating or calming these points, Shiatsu practitioners aim to enhance health and facilitate the body's natural healing abilities.

Thai Massage

Description: Thai massage, also known as "Thai yoga massage," combines acupressure, Indian Ayurvedic principles, and assisted yoga postures. It is a dynamic bodywork therapy that involves stretching and deep massage. Like Shiatsu, Thai massage is performed on a mat on the floor, and the recipient remains fully clothed. Practitioners use their body weight to increase the depth of the massage, utilizing their hands, knees, legs, and feet to move the recipient into a series of yoga-like stretches.

Theory: The theory behind Thai massage is also based on the concept of energy flow, similar to Shiatsu. However, it specifically focuses on the body's energy lines, known as "Sen" lines. Thai massage is designed to improve energy circulation, which is thought to be crucial for health and vitality. The practice believes in the concept of "Lom," which refers to wind or energy, and aims to release blockages along these lines, facilitating the body's natural healing processes. The stretching and massaging techniques employed in Thai massage are also intended to improve flexibility, relieve muscle and joint tension, and balance the body's energy systems.

While both Shiatsu and Thai massage are holistic practices designed to promote healing and balance within the body, they do so through different methodologies reflective of their cultural origins. Shiatsu focuses more on targeted pressure along meridian lines to directly influence the flow of Qi, while Thai massage incorporates a broader range of movements, including stretching and yoga-like postures, to work on the Sen lines and improve physical flexibility and energy flow.

Both forms of massage offer a deeply therapeutic experience, aiming to enhance physical, emotional, and spiritual well-being. The choice between them may depend on personal preference, specific health concerns, or the desired outcome of the therapy.

Chapter 6

Massage therapy offers a compassionate and holistic approach to addressing headaches and migraines, conditions that can significantly impact an individual's quality of life. This non-invasive treatment method focuses not only on relieving the immediate symptoms but also on understanding and addressing the underlying causes of the discomfort. By fostering a nurturing environment, massage therapy helps individuals find relief from the pain and stress associated with headaches and migraines.

Understanding Headaches and Migraines

Headaches and migraines can arise from a variety of factors, including stress, tension, dehydration, or underlying health issues. Migraines, in particular, are often accompanied by additional symptoms such as sensitivity to light, nausea, and visual disturbances. Both conditions can be debilitating, affecting an individual's ability to function normally in their daily life.

How Massage Therapy Helps

1. Reduction of Muscle Tension: One of the most common triggers for headaches, particularly tension headaches, is muscle stiffness and tension in the neck, shoulders, and scalp. Massage therapy directly addresses this by relaxing tight muscles, improving flexibility, and

decreasing pain. Techniques such as kneading and gentle stretching can significantly reduce the muscular tension that contributes to headache pain.

2. Stress Relief: Stress is a well-known trigger for both headaches and migraines. Massage therapy creates a peaceful, relaxing environment that encourages mental and emotional calm. This relaxation response can lower the body's production of stress hormones, which in turn can reduce the frequency and severity of headaches. The caring touch of a massage therapist can also promote a sense of being nurtured and cared for, which is especially comforting for those suffering from chronic conditions.

3. Improving Circulation: Enhanced blood flow is another benefit of massage therapy that can aid in headache relief. By improving circulation, massage can facilitate the delivery of oxygen and nutrients to tissues while helping to remove waste products. This improved blood flow can help alleviate the symptoms of headaches and support the body's natural healing processes.

4. Promoting Better Sleep: Poor sleep quality is both a contributor to and a result of migraines and headaches. Massage therapy can improve sleep patterns by promoting relaxation and reducing stress.

Better sleep can, in turn, reduce the likelihood of headache occurrences and contribute to overall well-being.

5. Holistic Approach: Massage therapists often take a holistic view of health, considering the physical, emotional, and lifestyle factors that may contribute to a person's headaches. By offering personalized care, they can provide recommendations for lifestyle adjustments, stress management techniques, and self-care practices that complement the physical benefits of massage.

Compassionate Care

For those experiencing headaches and migraines, the compassionate approach of massage therapy can be a beacon of hope. It offers not just a reduction in physical symptoms but also a moment of respite from the daily challenges posed by these conditions. The nurturing environment of massage therapy acknowledges the individual's experience of pain and seeks to provide relief in a caring, supportive manner.

Massage therapy addresses headaches and migraines with a compassionate touch, focusing on relieving tension, reducing stress, improving circulation, and fostering overall well-being. This holistic and nurturing approach provides a valuable complement to traditional medical treatments, offering a pathway to relief and comfort for those affected by these debilitating conditions.

Massage therapy can be a soothing and therapeutic approach for managing the symptoms of arthritis and fibromyalgia. Here's how it can help:

Massage helps in alleviating pain by improving circulation, which in turn reduces inflammation and promotes the healing of affected joints and muscles. This can be particularly beneficial for arthritis sufferers, as it helps reduce joint stiffness and discomfort. For those with arthritis, massage can aid in increasing flexibility and range of motion by relaxing and stretching the muscles surrounding the joints. This can lead to improved mobility and a decrease in the stiffness that often accompanies arthritis. Both arthritis and fibromyalgia can lead to significant stress and anxiety, partly due to chronic pain. Massage therapy promotes relaxation and releases tension, which can help lower stress levels. The reduction in stress can also positively affect the body's pain response, potentially leading to further relief from symptoms. Many individuals with fibromyalgia and arthritis struggle with sleep due to pain. Massage can encourage relaxation and increase serotonin levels, which may help improve sleep quality. Better sleep can further help in the healing and management of symptoms. Improved blood flow from massage can help reduce muscle spasms and increase oxygen and nutrients to the tissues. This can be particularly helpful for fibromyalgia patients, as increased circulation may help reduce the characteristic muscle pain and fatigue. Massage can aid in stimulating the lymphatic system, which helps in removing toxins from the body. This can contribute to a reduction in the swelling and inflammation often seen in arthritis.

It's important to note that while massage can provide relief, the level of benefit can vary from person to person. It's also crucial to consult with a healthcare provider before starting any new treatment to ensure it's safe and appropriate for your specific health condition. Additionally, finding a massage therapist experienced in working with arthritis and fibromyalgia patients can make a significant difference in the effectiveness of the therapy.

Massage therapy, when integrated into the compassionate care of cancer patients, can offer a multitude of benefits that support both physical and emotional well-being during an incredibly challenging time. Here's how massage plays a role in the compassionate care of those battling cancer:

Cancer and its treatments can lead to a variety of physical discomforts, including pain, nausea, and fatigue. Massage therapy can help alleviate some of these symptoms, offering a non-invasive form of relief. For example, gentle massage can reduce the intensity of pain, help manage stress, and improve relaxation, contributing to an overall sense of well-being.

The journey through cancer can be emotionally taxing. Massage provides a form of nurturing touch, which can be incredibly comforting. This compassionate contact can help reduce feelings of isolation, anxiety, and depression, offering emotional support and a sense of being cared for during a difficult time.

Studies have suggested that massage therapy can improve the quality of life for cancer patients by enhancing mood, improving sleep patterns, and reducing stress levels. These benefits are particularly important as they can help patients cope better with their diagnosis and treatments.

For patients who have undergone surgeries or treatments that affect the lymphatic system, certain types of massage, like manual lymph drainage, can help reduce lymphedema (swelling due to lymph fluid buildup). This can be crucial in managing one of the common side effects experienced by some cancer patients.

The stress and anxiety associated with cancer can make it difficult for patients to relax and sleep well. Massage therapy has been shown to promote relaxation and improve sleep patterns, which is vital for the healing process and overall quality of life.

Massage can help patients feel more connected to their bodies during a time when they might feel estranged from it due to illness and treatment. This connection can promote a sense of empowerment and body awareness, contributing to a more positive body image and self-esteem.

While massage therapy offers these benefits, it is crucial to approach it with care and consideration for the specific needs and medical conditions of each cancer patient. It's important to work with healthcare professionals and trained massage therapists who have experience in oncology massage. They can adapt massage techniques to ensure they are safe and appropriate for the patient's current condition, such as modifying pressure and avoiding direct massage on tumor sites or areas affected by radiation, chemotherapy ports, or medical device

In summary, massage therapy, as part of the compassionate care for cancer patients, provides a holistic approach that supports both the physical and emotional aspects of healing and coping with the disease.

Massage therapy during pregnancy can play a vital role in prenatal care, offering a range of benefits aimed at supporting the well-being of both the expectant mother and her baby. Here's how massage contributes to prenatal care:

Pregnancy can be a time of heightened emotions and anxiety about the health of the baby, the childbirth process, and the transition to parenthood. Massage therapy can help reduce stress levels through the release of endorphins, the body's natural feel-good hormones. This relaxation effect can also benefit the baby, as stress reduction in the mother has been linked to healthier pregnancy outcomes.

As the body changes to accommodate the growing fetus, discomforts such as backaches, stiff neck, leg cramps, headaches, and edema (swelling) can occur. Prenatal massage is tailored to an expectant mother's needs and can help relieve these discomforts by improving circulation, reducing muscle tension and inflammation, and enhancing the function of muscles and joints.

Many pregnant women experience difficulty sleeping due to discomfort, anxiety, or hormonal changes. Massage therapy can promote relaxation and improve sleep quality by soothing nervous system activity, making it easier for expectant mothers to rest and recuperate.

Improved blood flow from massage can provide more oxygen and nutrients to both the mother and the fetus. Additionally, enhanced circulation can help reduce swelling by assisting the lymphatic system in removing excess fluids and waste products from the body.

The nurturing touch of massage can provide emotional comfort and a sense of being cared for, which is especially important during the transformative period of pregnancy. This can help strengthen the emotional bond between the mother and her unborn child.

Some practitioners believe that regular prenatal massage can help prepare the mother's body for labor and delivery by promoting flexibility and readiness of the pelvic muscles. However, this is more about general relaxation and physical readiness than a direct effect on labor outcomes.

As the pregnancy progresses, the center of gravity shifts, often leading to posture adjustments that can cause muscle imbalances and pain. Massage can help address these imbalances by targeting specific muscle groups affected by these changes, providing relief and contributing to better posture.

It's important for pregnant women to consult with their healthcare provider before beginning any new therapy, including massage, to ensure it's safe for their specific situation. Additionally, finding a massage therapist trained in prenatal massage is crucial, as they will understand how to safely and effectively adjust their techniques to accommodate the needs of pregnant women, including proper positioning and avoiding certain pressure points that are contraindicated during pregnancy.

Prenatal massage is a supportive and beneficial component of comprehensive prenatal care, offering physical and emotional benefits that can enhance the pregnancy experience and potentially contribute to a healthier pregnancy and childbirth process.

Chapter 7

Finding a massage therapist who is a good fit for you involves several steps, aimed at ensuring that the therapist's qualifications, expertise, and approach align with your specific needs and preferences. Here's a step-by-step guide to help you in this process:

Before starting your search, clarify what you hope to achieve through massage therapy. Are you seeking relief from specific physical discomfort, such as back pain or muscle tension, or are you looking for general relaxation and stress reduction? Also, consider any preferences you have regarding the therapist's gender, the type of massage you're interested in (e.g., Swedish, deep tissue, prenatal), and any other factors that are important to you.

Look for therapists who have the appropriate certifications and qualifications. In many places, massage therapists are required to be licensed or certified, which involves completing an accredited program and passing a state or national exam. You can start your search by asking for referrals from healthcare providers, friends, or family members who have had positive experiences. Online directories and professional associations for massage therapists are also valuable resources.

Once you have a list of potential therapists, review their experience and areas of specialization. If you have a specific health condition or goal, like managing symptoms of a chronic illness or improving athletic performance, look for a therapist with expertise in that area. Many therapists list their qualifications, specializations, and approach on their websites or online profiles.

Reading reviews and testimonials from other clients can provide insights into the therapist's professionalism, approach, and the effectiveness of their treatments. While individual experiences can vary, patterns in feedback can be informative.

Many therapists offer a brief consultation, either over the phone or in person, at no charge. Use this opportunity to ask about their approach, techniques, experience with clients who have needs similar to yours, and how they tailor their sessions to individual clients. This is also a good time to discuss any concerns or questions you have.

A good massage therapist will ask about your health history, your goals for massage therapy, and any specific concerns or conditions you have. This conversation helps ensure that the therapy is safe and tailored to your needs. If a therapist does not ask about your health history or seems dismissive of your concerns, it may be a sign to look elsewhere.

Feeling comfortable with your massage therapist is crucial. Pay attention to how well they communicate with you, respect your boundaries, and address your comfort and concerns. The therapist should make you feel heard and respected and provide a safe, comfortable environment.

If you're unsure, consider booking a single session to evaluate the experience. This can help you decide if the therapist's style, pressure, and approach are a good fit for you without making a long-term commitment.

After your session, reflect on how you felt during and after the massage. Consider whether your needs were met, how your body responded to the therapy, and whether you felt comfortable and respected by the therapist.

Ultimately, the right therapist for you is one with whom you feel a sense of trust and comfort, and who can effectively address your specific needs and goals for massage therapy.

Remember, finding the right massage therapist might take some time and experimentation, but the benefits of finding a good match for your needs can significantly enhance your overall well-being and therapy experience.

Tailoring a massage plan to an individual's needs is a thoughtful process that involves understanding the person's health history, current physical condition, goals for massage therapy, and personal preferences. Here's a guide on how to create a personalized massage plan:

Start with a detailed intake form that asks about the client's medical history, any current health conditions, areas of pain or discomfort, lifestyle factors (such as activity level and stress), and what they hope to achieve through massage therapy. This information is crucial for designing a safe and effective massage plan.

Before the first session, conduct a consultation to discuss the information provided in the intake form. This is also an opportunity to assess posture, range of motion, and any specific areas of tension or discomfort. The assessment can be both verbal, asking about areas of concern, and physical, through observation and gentle palpation.

Based on the intake and assessment, work with the client to set clear, achievable goals for the massage therapy. Goals can range from reducing pain in a specific area, improving flexibility, reducing stress and anxiety, enhancing sleep quality, or addressing specific conditions like headaches or repetitive strain injuries.

Select massage techniques and modalities that align with the client's goals, health status, and preferences. For example, a client with chronic muscle tension may benefit from deep tissue massage, while someone seeking relaxation and stress reduction may prefer Swedish massage. Consider also the use of adjunct therapies like hot stone therapy, aromatherapy, or reflexology if appropriate and desired by the client.

Decide on the frequency, duration, and structure of the sessions. This includes how much time will be spent on each area of the body and which areas require special attention. The plan should be flexible, allowing adjustments based on the client's feedback and progress.

Tailor the environment and the session to the client's comfort and preferences. This includes room temperature, lighting, music, and the use of cushions or supports to ensure comfort throughout the massage.

Encourage open communication during and after the sessions, asking for feedback on the pressure and techniques used. After each session, discuss any changes in the client's condition or goals and adjust the massage plan accordingly.

Regularly reassess the client's progress towards their goals, adjusting the massage plan as needed. This may involve changing techniques, focusing on different areas of the body, or altering the frequency of sessions.

Provide the client with information and resources that can help them maintain or enhance the benefits of massage between sessions. This might include stretches, posture tips, stress management strategies, or lifestyle adjustments.

Keep detailed records of each session, including techniques used, client feedback, progress towards goals, and any adjustments made to the plan. This documentation is essential for tracking the client's progress and making informed decisions about future sessions.

Tailoring a massage plan requires a balance of professional expertise, empathy, and open communication. By focusing on the individual's unique needs and goals, a massage therapist can create a personalized approach that maximizes the therapeutic benefits and enhances the overall well-being of the client.

Integrating massage into a general wellness routine is a holistic approach to maintaining and enhancing overall health. Massage therapy complements other wellness practices by addressing physical, emotional, and mental health components. Here's how massage can be integrated into a broader wellness strategy:

Regular massage sessions can significantly reduce stress levels, which is a critical component of overall wellness. By lowering cortisol levels and increasing serotonin and dopamine levels, massage promotes relaxation and improves mood, helping to mitigate the negative effects of stress on the body.

Massage therapy can enhance physical wellness by improving circulation, reducing muscle tension and pain, increasing flexibility and range of motion, and stimulating the lymphatic system to aid in detoxification. These benefits can support more active lifestyles and make other forms of exercise more enjoyable and less painful.

The relaxation and stress relief provided by massage can have profound effects on mental health. By promoting a state of calm and relaxation, massage can help alleviate symptoms of anxiety and depression, contributing to a more balanced and positive mental state.

Regular massage can improve sleep quality by promoting relaxation and reducing pain and discomfort that might interfere with sleep. Better sleep contributes to overall health by aiding in recovery, improving immune function, and enhancing mental health.

For individuals managing chronic conditions or recovering from injuries, massage can be a valuable complement to medical care. It can help manage symptoms, reduce pain, and improve recovery outcomes when integrated into a treatment plan with the guidance of healthcare professionals.

Massage encourages individuals to focus on the present moment and increases body awareness. This mindfulness can enhance the connection between the mind and body, encouraging more mindful eating, exercise, and lifestyle choices that contribute to overall wellness.

Massage therapy works synergistically with other components of a wellness routine, such as physical exercise, yoga, meditation, and balanced nutrition. For example, massage can enhance the benefits of yoga and exercise by improving flexibility and reducing muscle soreness, making these activities more effective and enjoyable.

How to Integrate Massage into Your Wellness Routine:

Regular Scheduling: Incorporate regular massage sessions into your wellness routine, much like you would exercise or meditation. This regularity helps maintain the cumulative benefits of massage over time.

Personalized Approach: Choose massage types and frequencies that align with your wellness goals and preferences. For example, if stress reduction is a priority, you might opt for Swedish massage or aromatherapy massage.

Holistic Wellness Plan: Consider massage as part of a broader wellness plan that includes physical activity, proper nutrition, hydration, and sufficient rest. Consult with wellness professionals to create a balanced and comprehensive plan.

Listen to Your Body: Use massage as a way to tune into your body's needs and responses. It can be a tool for identifying areas of tension or imbalance that might need attention in your wellness routine.

Mindfulness and Relaxation: Use the time during massage to practice mindfulness or meditation, enhancing the mental and emotional benefits of both the massage and your overall wellness routine.

Integrating massage into your wellness routine offers a multi-faceted approach to health that supports the body, mind, and spirit. By making massage a regular part of your wellness practice, you can enhance your ability to manage stress, maintain physical health, and cultivate a more balanced and healthy lifestyle.

Chapter 8

Practicing basic self-massage is a wonderful way to relieve tension, reduce stress, and promote relaxation in your own comfort space. Here's a simple guide to get you started with basic self-massage techniques that can be easily incorporated into your daily routine:

1. Hand Massage:

Technique: Start by applying a lotion or oil to your hands to reduce friction. Use the thumb of one hand to make circular motions on the palm of the other hand, working your way from the center to the outer edges. Next, gently pull each finger from the base to the tip, twisting slightly as you go. This can help relieve tension from typing or other manual tasks.

2. Neck and Shoulder Massage:

Technique: Gently squeeze the shoulders with the opposite hand, moving from the base of your neck to the edge of your shoulder. Use your fingertips to make small, circular motions along the neck and the base of the skull. Tilting your head from side to side as you massage can help extend the area of relief.

3. Foot Massage:

Technique: Sit comfortably and place one foot over the opposite knee. Use your hands to rub the entire foot, applying gentle pressure with your thumbs to the bottom of the foot, moving in circular motions. Pay special attention to the arches and the balls of the feet, which can accumulate a lot of tension.

4. Arm and Forearm Massage:

Technique: With one hand, grasp the opposite arm and squeeze gently, working your way from the elbow down to the wrist and then back up. Use your thumb to apply more focused pressure in circular motions on the forearm, which can be particularly soothing if you experience tension from computer work.

5. Lower Back Massage:

Technique: Place a tennis ball or a similar object between your lower back and a wall. Lean into the ball and slowly move your body up, down, and side to side, allowing the ball to massage any tense areas. Be gentle and avoid putting pressure directly on the spine.

6. Head and Scalp Massage:

Technique: Place the fingertips of both hands on your scalp. Apply gentle pressure and move your fingers in small circular motions, covering the entire head. This can be incredibly relaxing and may also help relieve headaches.

Tips for Effective Self-Massage:

Relax and Breathe: Before starting, take a few deep breaths to relax. Continue to breathe deeply and slowly during your self-massage to enhance relaxation.

Mindful Attention: Pay attention to how each part of your body feels as you massage it. Adjust the pressure to what feels good; it should never cause pain.

Consistency: Regularly incorporating self-massage into your routine can yield more lasting benefits, such as reduced stress and improved circulation.

Comfortable Setting: Create a calming environment by dimming the lights, playing soft music, or using essential oils to enhance the relaxation experience.

Self-massage is a flexible and accessible tool that can significantly contribute to your overall well-being. By regularly practicing these simple techniques, you can effectively manage stress, relieve tension, and promote a sense of calm and relaxation in your daily life.

Partner massage can be a wonderful way to connect, provide comfort, and help each other relax. It's a mutual exchange of trust and care, allowing both partners to experience the benefits of massage without the need for professional training. Here are some techniques that are particularly effective and easy to apply in a partner massage setting:

Effleurage (Gentle Stroking)

Description: This technique involves light, gentle strokes over the skin, using the palms and fingertips. It's often used to begin and end the massage session because it soothes and relaxes.

Application: Start with your hands on your partner's shoulders or back. Gently glide your hands down their body in a smooth, flowing motion, applying light pressure. Repeat with slow, rhythmic strokes to help your partner relax.

Petrissage (Kneading):

Description: Petrissage involves deeper, circular movements using the fingers and palms. It's designed to work deeper tissues, improving circulation and relieving muscle tension.

Application: After warming up the muscles with effleurage, use your hands to gently lift, squeeze, and press the muscles, especially in areas like the shoulders, upper arms, and legs. Imagine you're kneading dough, but be mindful of your partner's comfort level regarding pressure.

Thumb Circles:

Description: This technique uses the thumbs to apply pressure in small circles, targeting specific areas of tension.

Application: Identify areas of tightness or knots, and use your thumbs to gently make small, circular movements. This is particularly effective for the neck, shoulders, and back. Adjust the pressure based on your partner's feedback, ensuring it's firm but comfortable.

Compression:

Description: Compression involves applying direct pressure with the hands, elbows, or forearms to various parts of the body. This helps to relax tight muscles and improve blood flow.

Application: Use the heel of your hand or your forearm to apply steady, direct pressure to areas like the back, thighs, or calves. Lean into the movement using your body weight to control the pressure, but be careful not to apply too much force.

Gliding Forearm Strokes:

Description: This technique uses the broad surface of the forearm to apply pressure over a larger area, providing a deep sense of relaxation and stress relief.

Application: Place your forearm on a large muscle group, such as the back or thigh. Apply gentle pressure and glide your forearm up and down or across the muscle, allowing the natural weight of your arm to do the work.

Tips for Partner Massage:

Communicate: Keep the lines of communication open. Ask your partner for feedback on the pressure and technique, and adjust accordingly.

Create a Relaxing Environment: Dim the lights, play soft music, and ensure the room is a comfortable temperature.

Use Massage Oil or Lotion: This reduces friction and makes the massage more enjoyable. Warm the oil or lotion in your hands before applying it to your partner's skin.

Be Mindful of Your Own Comfort: Adjust your posture and position to ensure you're comfortable throughout the massage. This will help you maintain consistent pressure and prevent strain on your own body.

Remember, the goal of partner massage is to relax and connect with each other. There's no need to aim for professional perfection. Instead, focus on the intention of care and the enjoyment of sharing a peaceful, relaxing experience together.

Incorporating tools and products into a massage session can significantly enhance the experience, making it more relaxing, therapeutic, and enjoyable. Here's an overview of various items that can be used and how they contribute to an enhanced massage experience:

Massage Oils and Lotions

Purpose: Reduce friction on the skin, allowing for smoother, more comfortable massage strokes. They can also nourish the skin, leaving it soft and hydrated.

Types: There are many types of massage oils and lotions to choose from, including almond oil, coconut oil, jojoba oil, and shea butter lotion. Each has its own benefits and suitability for different skin types.

Essential Oils

Purpose: When used in aromatherapy massage, essential oils can promote relaxation, relieve stress, and improve mood. Each essential oil has its own therapeutic properties.

Examples:

Lavender: Known for its calming and relaxing properties.

Peppermint: Refreshing and can help relieve muscle pain.

Eucalyptus: Soothing for respiratory issues and provides a cooling sensation.

Rosemary: Stimulating, helps improve circulation and relieve muscle aches.

Hot Stones

Purpose: Hot stone massage involves placing warmed stones on certain areas of the body. The heat from the stones penetrates deeply into the muscles, helping to relieve tension, ease sore muscles, and enhance relaxation.

Application: Stones are typically heated in water and then placed along the spine, in the palms, or even between toes. The therapist may also use the stones as an extension of their hands while massaging.

Massage Tools

Purpose: Various tools can be used to apply pressure or massage certain areas of the body, often allowing for deeper pressure or targeted relief.

Examples:

Foam rollers: Used for self-massage to release muscle tightness or trigger points.

Massage balls: Ideal for targeting specific areas, such as under the feet or the back.

Electric massagers: Offer vibration or percussion therapy to help relax muscles and relieve pain.

Massage Tables and Chairs

Purpose: Provide a comfortable and supportive surface for the person receiving the massage.

Details: A good massage table or chair is adjustable and cushioned, making it easier to access and effectively massage all areas of the body while ensuring comfort for the client.

Towels and Blankets

Purpose: Ensure privacy, comfort, and warmth during the massage. They can also be used to drape and support the body in certain positions.

Application: Soft, fluffy towels and blankets can enhance the sense of luxury and relaxation during the massage.

Music and Lighting

Purpose: Create a relaxing and inviting atmosphere that complements the physical benefits of the massage.

Details: Soft, ambient music and dim, warm lighting can help soothe the mind and enhance the overall massage experience.

Using These Tools and Products

When incorporating these tools and products into a massage, it's essential to consider the individual's preferences, allergies, or sensitivities, particularly with essential oils and lotions. Always conduct a patch test with new products and discuss any health concerns or preferences with the person receiving the massage.

By thoughtfully selecting and integrating these elements into a massage session, you can create a deeply relaxing, therapeutic, and personalized experience that nourishes the body, mind, and spirit.

Chapter 9

Massage therapy, despite its growing popularity and recognition as a valuable component of holistic health and wellness, is still subject to misconceptions and fears. Understanding and addressing these concerns is crucial for both practitioners and those considering massage therapy. Here are some common misconceptions and fears, along with analyses to help clarify and dispel them:

Misconception: Massage is Only for Relaxation and Luxury

Analysis: While massage is widely recognized for its ability to promote relaxation and is often associated with spa settings, its benefits extend far beyond. Massage therapy can be an effective treatment for a range of physical conditions, including muscle pain, tension, chronic pain management, and rehabilitation from injuries. It also has psychological benefits, helping to reduce symptoms of anxiety and depression.

Fear: Massage Therapy Can Be Painful

Analysis: Some people fear that massage therapy, especially types like deep tissue massage, will be painful. While some discomfort can be expected when addressing deep-set tension or knots, a skilled massage therapist will work within the client's comfort threshold and communicate openly about pressure levels. The goal is to relieve tension and pain, not cause it.

Misconception: Massage is Not Safe for Everyone

Analysis: This misconception may stem from a lack of understanding of the different types of massage and the ability to tailor sessions to individual needs and conditions. While there are contraindications for certain health conditions (e.g., certain stages of pregnancy, specific injuries, or illnesses), a qualified therapist can adjust their techniques and approaches to ensure safety and benefits for almost everyone.

Fear: Need to Be Completely Undressed

Analysis: The idea of undressing can be uncomfortable for many. However, clients are typically asked to undress to their level of comfort and are draped with sheets or towels to maintain privacy throughout the session. Only the part of the body being worked on is uncovered at any time.

Misconception: All Massage is the Same

Analysis: There's a wide variety of massage techniques and styles, each with different methods, purposes, and benefits. These range from gentle styles like Swedish massage to more intense forms like sports massage or trigger point therapy. Therapists can customize the session based on the client's specific needs and preferences.

Fear: Being Judged on Body Shape or Size

Analysis: Some individuals may hesitate to seek massage therapy due to self-consciousness or fear of judgment about their body. Professional massage therapists are trained to treat clients with respect and confidentiality, focusing on their well-being without judgment regarding body shape, size, conditions, or scars.

Misconception: Massage Therapy is Unregulated

Analysis: This varies by location, but in many regions, massage therapists are required to undergo extensive training, adhere to professional standards, and obtain licensure or certification. This regulatory framework ensures that therapists have the necessary qualifications and adhere to ethical practices.

Addressing These Misconceptions and Fears:

Educating the public about the diverse types of massage, their benefits, and the professional standards governing the field is vital. It's also important for therapists to communicate openly with clients, addressing any concerns or fears they may have and explaining the processes, techniques, and safety measures involved in massage therapy. By doing so, potential clients can be more informed and feel more comfortable about incorporating massage therapy into their wellness routines.

Massage therapy offers numerous benefits, including stress relief, pain reduction, and improved circulation, among others. However, there are contraindications and limitations to be aware of, ensuring the safety and well-being of individuals seeking massage therapy. Understanding these helps in making informed decisions about when to avoid or modify massage therapy sessions.

Contraindications of Massage

1. Acute Injuries or Inflammation: Massage directly on or near areas of acute injury, inflammation, or swelling is contraindicated, as it can exacerbate the condition. This includes recent fractures, burns, cuts, and bruises.

2. **Infectious Diseases:** Individuals with infectious diseases, including the flu or tuberculosis, should avoid massage as it can spread the infection, both through close contact and by taxing the immune system.

3. **Cardiovascular Conditions:** Those with severe cardiovascular conditions, such as thrombosis, phlebitis, or recent heart attacks, should exercise caution. Massage can increase circulation, potentially dislodging blood clots.

4. Skin Conditions: Open wounds, rashes, or infectious skin diseases like fungal infections, herpes, or shingles are contraindications for massage. Direct contact can irritate skin conditions or spread the infection.

5. Severe Osteoporosis: Individuals with severe osteoporosis or bone fractures from cancer may be at risk for injury from certain massage techniques.

6. Pregnancy: While prenatal massage can be beneficial, certain pressure points are believed to induce labor and should be avoided. It's essential to seek a therapist trained in prenatal massage.

7. Cancer: People undergoing cancer treatment or with cancerous tumors should consult their healthcare provider. While massage can be beneficial for relaxation and symptom relief, certain considerations must be made, such as avoiding direct pressure over tumor sites.

Limitations of Massage

1. Not a Substitute for Medical Treatment: While massage can complement medical treatment, it should not replace conventional care for serious health conditions. It's crucial for individuals with chronic or serious health issues to consult healthcare professionals before undergoing massage therapy.

2. Temporary Relief: Massage can provide significant relief from symptoms like muscle tension and stress. However, the effects are often temporary, requiring regular sessions for sustained benefits.

3. Variability in Practitioner Skill and Experience: The effectiveness of massage can greatly depend on the skill and experience of the therapist. Practitioners vary in their expertise with different conditions and techniques, affecting outcomes.

4. Subjectivity of Comfort and Experience: Personal preferences play a significant role in the massage experience. What is relaxing and therapeutic for one person may not be for another, affecting the perceived effectiveness of the therapy.

5. Cost and Accessibility: Regular massage sessions can be costly and may not be covered by health insurance. This can limit access for some individuals who might benefit from regular sessions.

Addressing Contraindications and Limitations

To mitigate risks and enhance the benefits of massage, it's important for therapists to conduct a thorough intake process, understanding a client's medical history, current health status, and goals for massage therapy. Clients should be encouraged to communicate openly about their comfort and any adverse reactions they experience during or after sessions.

In cases where massage is contraindicated, therapists can offer alternative methods of care or adjustments to the massage technique to accommodate the individual's needs safely. Collaboration with healthcare providers can also ensure that massage therapy is integrated appropriately into the individual's overall care plan.

Understanding and respecting the contraindications and limitations of massage therapy is essential for both therapists and clients to ensure that massage remains a safe and beneficial part of wellness and healthcare routines.

Conclusion

Let's lighten things up a bit with a humorous take on the benefits of massage therapy:

Stress Melt-Away Magic: Ever felt like a tightly wound spring, ready to snap at the slightest provocation? Well, massage is like that magical spell that turns you from a tense troll back into your charming self. It's the closest thing we have to a "chill pill."

Muscle Whisperer: Those knots in your muscles are like stubborn little gremlins, refusing to leave. Enter massage therapy: the muscle whisperer. It sweet-talks those knots into submission, leaving your muscles as relaxed as a cat in a sunbeam.

Circulation Circus: If your blood flow is more like a lazy river than a lively stream, massage therapy kicks it into gear. Think of it as the ringmaster, getting the circulation show on the road, ensuring every part of you gets a ticket to the nutrient and oxygen party.

Detox Dance-Off: Massage gets your lymphatic system grooving, helping your body to kick toxins to the curb. It's like inviting your organs to a dance-off, where the prize is feeling fabulous and detoxified.

Flexibility Festival: Feeling more like the Tin Man than a bendy straw? Massage therapy is your ticket to the flexibility festival, helping you bend and stretch with the best of them. Yoga poses you once dreamed of mastering suddenly become part of your morning routine.

Sleep Serenade: If counting sheep has become a nightly ritual, a massage might just be the lullaby you need. It serenades your nervous system into a state of blissful relaxation, helping you catch those elusive Z's.

Mood Makeover: In a grump slump? Massage therapy can give your mood a makeover, turning those frowns upside down. It's like having a personal cheerleader for your serotonin and dopamine levels, ensuring you feel more "yay" than "nay."

Pain's Nemesis: Chronic pain got you feeling like a villain in your own comic book? Massage is the superhero swooping in to save the day, tackling pain and leaving you feeling like you've got a new lease on life.

So, there you have it—a whimsical whirlwind tour through the wonderland of massage therapy benefits. It's not just a treat for the body but a feast for the soul, and possibly the best "me-time" you can schedule that doesn't involve Netflix. Remember, a good laugh and a long massage are two of the best cures in the doctor's book!

Embarking on a journey with massage therapy as a complementary practice is like opening the door to a treasure trove of wellness wonders. Imagine having a tool at your disposal that not only soothes the body but also calms the mind and nourishes the soul—massage is that tool, wrapped in a bow of tranquility and tied with strings of rejuvenation.

Diving into the world of massage therapy, you're not just exploring a range of techniques; you're embracing an ancient tradition that has comforted and healed humanity through centuries. From the gentle, flowing strokes of Swedish massage to the targeted pressure of deep tissue work, each modality offers its own unique path to balance and well-being.

Think of massage as your personal oasis in the desert of daily life—a sanctuary where stress is a distant memory, and peace is the order of the day. It's a chance to tune out the noise, to listen to the whispers of your body, and to honor its needs with kindness and care.

For those a tad wary of stepping into this new territory, let curiosity be your guide. The beauty of massage lies in its adaptability to your individual needs and comfort levels. There's a vast spectrum of styles and techniques, ensuring that there's something for everyone, whether you're seeking relief from chronic pain, looking to reduce stress, or simply aiming to maintain a harmonious balance between body and mind.

Remember, embarking on this journey doesn't mean leaving behind conventional medical care. Instead, it's about enriching your wellness toolkit, adding layers of depth to your self-care regimen, and discovering holistic paths to health that complement the care you receive from your healthcare provider.

So, why not take that first step? Your body, with all its wisdom and wonder, deserves to be cherished. Massage therapy offers a bridge to deeper understanding and connection with your own physical being, opening doors to improved health, enhanced well-being, and joy in the simple luxury of feeling good.

Let this be your invitation to explore, to experience, and to embrace the myriad benefits that massage therapy can bring into your life. The journey toward wellness is a personal adventure, and massage is a companion worth considering on your path to a happier, healthier you.

The future of massage therapy is on an exciting trajectory, evolving through innovations in technology, deeper integration with healthcare, and a growing recognition of its holistic benefits. As we look forward, several key trends and developments suggest a dynamic expansion of massage therapy's role in wellness and medicine.

Integration with Healthcare Systems

Massage therapy is increasingly being recognized as a valuable complementary therapy within conventional healthcare settings. This trend is expected to grow, with more doctors and healthcare providers recommending massage as part of treatment plans for a variety of conditions, from chronic pain management to recovery from injuries and surgeries. The integration is facilitated by a growing body of research that validates the efficacy of massage therapy in alleviating symptoms and improving patient outcomes.

Personalization Through Technology

Technology is set to play a significant role in the evolution of massage therapy. Wearable devices and mobile apps that track stress levels, posture, and muscle tension in real-time can provide data-driven insights into an individual's specific needs, allowing for highly personalized massage therapies. Additionally, advancements in tools and equipment, such as smart massage tables and devices that can simulate various massage techniques, could enhance the effectiveness of treatments and accessibility for home use.

Specialization and Advanced Training

As the field grows, there is an increasing trend towards specialization among massage therapists. Professionals are seeking advanced training in areas such as sports massage, oncology massage, and neuromuscular therapy, among others. This specialization allows therapists to offer more targeted and effective treatments for specific conditions, appealing to a broader range of clients seeking relief for particular health issues.

Holistic and Preventative Approach

There is a growing awareness of the preventative benefits of massage therapy, not just as a remedy for existing conditions but as a routine practice to maintain overall health and well-being. This holistic approach views massage as an integral part of a preventative healthcare regimen, encouraging regular sessions to manage stress, enhance immune function, improve sleep, and maintain physical and mental well-being.

Virtual Reality and Augmented Reality

Emerging technologies like virtual reality (VR) and augmented reality (AR) could transform the massage experience, offering immersive environments that enhance relaxation and stress relief. Imagine a massage session where you're visually transported to a tranquil beach or a serene forest; these technologies could amplify the therapeutic effects of massage by engaging the senses more fully.

Collaboration with Mental Health

The link between physical touch and mental health is well-documented, and the future may see massage therapy playing a more prominent role in mental health treatment plans. By reducing stress and anxiety, massage can be an effective complement to psychotherapy and other mental health interventions, offering a holistic approach to mental wellness.

Sustainability and Ethical Practices

As society becomes more environmentally conscious, the demand for sustainable and ethically sourced massage products (oils, creams, tables) is rising. Massage therapists and businesses will likely place greater emphasis on using organic, cruelty-free, and sustainably produced products, aligning with the values of environmentally conscious consumers.

Looking ahead, the future of massage therapy is bright, marked by deeper integration with healthcare, technological advancements, and a growing appreciation for its holistic benefits. This evolution reflects a broader shift towards more personalized, preventative, and holistic approaches to health and wellness, ensuring massage therapy's vital place in the wellness landscape of tomorrow.